ACRONYMS

CBOC	Community Based Outpatient Clinic
ECHCS	Eastern Colorado Health Care System
HAS	Health Administration Service
NVCC	Non-VA Care Coordination
OIG	Office of Inspector General
VA	Department of Veterans Affairs
VACAA	Veterans Access, Choice, and Accountability Act of 2014
VAMC	VA Medical Center
VCL	Veterans Choice List
VCP	Veterans Choice Program
VHA	Veterans Health Administration

To Report Suspected Wrongdoing in VA Programs and Operations:

Telephone: 1-800-488-8244

E-Mail: vaoighotline@va.gov

(Hotline Information: http://www.va.gov/oig/hotline)

Report Highlights: Review of Alleged Untimely Care at VHA's Community Based Outpatient Clinic Colorado Springs, CO

Why We Did This Review

In January 2015, the Office of Inspector General received an allegation that the PFC Floyd K. Lindstrom Outpatient Clinic, a Community Based Outpatient Clinic (CBOC) in Colorado Springs, CO, did not provide veterans' access to the Veterans Choice Program when the CBOC did not provide veterans timely VA care. One affected veteran sent the complaint, along with examples of issues affecting clinic services provided in audiology, mental health, neurology, optometry, orthopedic, and primary care.

What We Found

We substantiated the allegation that the veteran, as well as other eligible Colorado Springs veterans, did not receive timely care in the six reviewed services. We reviewed 150 referrals for specialty care consults and 300 primary care appointments. Of the 450 consults and appointments, 288 veterans encountered wait times in excess of 30 days. For all 288 veterans, VA staff either did not add them to the Veterans Choice List (VCL) or did not add them to the VCL in a timely manner.

For 59 of the 288 veterans, scheduling staff used incorrect dates that made it appear the appointment wait time was less than 30 days. For 229 of the 288 veterans with appointments over 30 days, NVCC staff did not add 173 veterans at the CBOCs in the Eastern Colorado Health Care System (ECHCS) to the VCL in a timely manner and they did not add 56 veterans to the list at all. In addition, scheduling staff did not take timely action on 94 consults and primary care appointment requests. As a result, VA staff did not fully use Veterans Choice Program funds to afford CBOC Colorado Springs veterans the opportunity to receive timely care.

What We Recommended

We recommended that the ECHCS Director take actions to ensure appointments are scheduled using clinically indicated or preferred appointment dates, all veterans eligible for the Veterans Choice Program are added to the VCL in a timely manner, and scheduling staff timely act on consults and appointment requests.

Management Comments

The acting director of the ECHCS concurred in principle with our recommendations. ECHCS executed a number of corrective actions to become compliant with current VHA scheduling guidance. Based on actions already implemented, we consider Recommendation 1 closed. We will follow up on the implementation of the remaining recommendations until all proposed actions are completed.

GARY K. ABE
Acting Assistant Inspector General
for Audits and Evaluations

TABLE OF CONTENTS

Results and Recommendations 1

    Allegation   Were Colorado Springs Veterans Provided Access to the Veterans
                     Choice Program When Timely VA Care Was Not Provided? 1

                     Recommendations 8

    Appendix A   Background 10

    Appendix B   Scope and Methodology 12

    Appendix C   Eastern Colorado Health Care System Director Comments 14

    Appendix D   OIG Contact and Staff Acknowledgments....................................... 18

    Appendix E   Report Distribution..19

RESULTS AND RECOMMENDATIONS

Allegation

Were Colorado Springs Veterans Provided Access to the Veterans Choice Program When Timely VA Care Was Not Provided?

On January 26, 2015, the Office of Inspector General (OIG) received an allegation that the PFC Floyd K. Lindstrom Outpatient Clinic, a Community Based Outpatient Clinic (CBOC) in Colorado Springs, CO, did not provide veterans' access to the Veterans Choice Program (VCP) when the Eastern Colorado Health Care System (ECHCS) did not provide veterans timely VA care. The veteran who sent the complaint provided examples about his experiences with Audiology, Mental Health, Neurology, Optometry, Orthopedic, and Primary Care Services.

The CBOC Colorado Springs is 1 of 10 community clinics in the ECHCS. The CBOC provides primary and some specialty care services to veterans in the Colorado Springs area. Specialty care includes audiology, dental, mental health, optometry, and substance abuse services. The CBOC refers patients to the VA Medical Center (VAMC) in Denver, CO for neurology and orthopedic services.

Assessment

We substantiated that for 450 consults and appointments we reviewed, 288 (64 percent) Colorado Springs veterans did not receive timely care in the Audiology, Mental Health, Neurology, Optometry, Orthopedic, and Primary Care Services. Staff either did not add them to the Veterans Choice List (VCL) or did not add them in a timely manner. This occurred because scheduling staff used incorrect clinically indicated or preferred appointment dates, Non-VA Care Coordination (NVCC) staff did not properly manage the VCL, and scheduling staff did not take action on consults and appointments in a timely manner.

What We Did

We interviewed CBOC Colorado Springs and VAMC Denver staff, physicians, and program managers to assess the merits of the allegation. We also interviewed the complainant to gain a full understanding of the allegations. To understand the policy implementation of Veterans Access, Choice, and Availability Act of 2014 (VACAA), we interviewed the Chief Business Officer, Chief Business Office staff, and VA Central Office program officials responsible for Veterans Health Administration's (VHA) appointment and consult management guidance. We reviewed the processes for scheduling consults, identifying availability of appointments for providers, and adding veterans to the VCL. To evaluate the timeliness of care, we reviewed data in the VHA Support Service Center and the Compensation and Pension Records Interchange systems.

Appointments Were Scheduled Over 30 Days

We identified 288 veterans from the 450 consults and appointments (64 percent) we reviewed who encountered wait times in excess of 30 days consisting of:

- *Specialty Care Consult*—We reviewed 150 specialty care consults. Of these, 54 (36 percent) were for veterans who had appointments scheduled to occur more than 30 days from the consult request date and had an average wait time of 66 days—ranging from 31 to 148 days.

- *Primary Care Appointments*—We reviewed 300 primary care appointments. Of these, 234 (78 percent) were for veterans who had appointments scheduled to occur more than 30 days from the clinically indicated or preferred appointment dates and had an average wait time of 68 days—ranging from 32 to 229 days.

According to VCP implementation guidance, VA has a wait time goal to furnish care within 30 days or staff are required to place the veteran on the VCL. VA calculates the 30 days from the appropriate date of care to the appointment date. The appropriate date of care for an appointment entered into the scheduling system is the provider's clinically indicated date, earliest appropriate date as indicated on a consult for new patient referrals, or a date the patient requests (preferred date). According to VA's terms with the VCP contractors, VA staff will provide a daily list of veterans eligible for inclusion on the VCL because they have appointments scheduled beyond 30 days from the clinically indicated or preferred appointment date. The contractors use this information to schedule the necessary care.

We compared the VCL, dated August 11, 2015, with the list of 288 veterans to determine if they were on the VCL. If they were, we determined whether VA staff added them within a day of creating the appointment. NVCC staff did not add, or did not timely add, the 288 veterans with appointments scheduled more than 30 days beyond the clinically indicated or preferred appointment dates of care.

Table 1 shows the numbers of veterans whom NVCC staff did not add to the VCL, or did not timely add to the VCL, for each of the services reviewed.

Table 1. Delays in Care and Untimely Placement on the VCL

Clinic	Number of Appointments Reviewed	Veterans With Appointments Beyond 30 Days	Veterans Not on VCL	Veterans on VCL, but Not Timely Added
Audiology Consults	30	21	10	11
Mental Health Consults	30	3	3	0
Neurology Consults	30	10	8	2
Optometry Consults	30	17	12	5
Orthopedic Consults	30	3	3	0
Consults Subtotal	**150**	**54**	**36**	**18**
Primary Care Appointments	300	234	64	170
Total Consults and Appointments	**450**	**288**	**100**	**188**

Source: VA OIG Analysis of Data in the Compensation and Pension Records Interchange System for the Denver VA Medical Center

For the veterans not added to the VCL timely, the average delay for Audiology, Neurology, Optometry, and Primary Care clinics was 44, 30, 39, and 46 days, respectively. The minimum delay for adding a veteran to the VCL was 4 days for a patient in the Optometry clinic and the maximum delay was 189 days for a patient in a primary care clinic.

Scheduling Staff Used Incorrect Dates

For 59 of the 288 veterans with appointments more than 30 days, scheduling staff used incorrect dates that made it appear the appointment wait time was less than 30 days. Of these 59 appointments scheduled more than 30 days from the clinically indicated or preferred appointment dates, 34 were for primary care appointments and 25 were for appointments scheduled from consults.

Primary Care Appointments

Scheduling staff used incorrect clinically indicated or preferred appointment dates for 34 primary care appointments that resulted in NVCC staff leaving veterans off the VCL even though these veterans waited more than 30 days for their appointment.

- For 28 of these 34 primary care appointments, scheduling staff identified the first available appointment and then used that date as the preferred date of care. This practice resulted in appointments that showed an incorrect zero-day wait time. In actuality, these 28 veterans waited an average of 72 days—ranging from 32 to 160 days for their initial primary care appointments.

- For 6 of the 34 primary care appointments, scheduling staff incorrectly used the date they created the appointment for newly enrolled veterans instead of using the appointment request date, which was weeks earlier. These veterans waited an average of 76 days—ranging from 32 to 157 days—for their initial primary care appointments.

Example 1 shows the effect of staff's incorrect use of the veteran's preferred appointment date on the appointment's wait time.

Example 1

An Operation Enduring Freedom/Operation Iraqi Freedom veteran had an initial intake assessment performed on November 13, 2014, when the veteran indicated he wanted an appointment with a primary care provider. Staff scheduled a primary care appointment for the veteran on January 29, 2015, which was 77 days later. However, according to the Health Administration Service (HAS) Chief, the scheduler incorrectly used the appointment date as the veteran's preferred date, which resulted in an erroneous zero-day wait time. The HAS Chief agreed that the scheduler should not have used the appointment date as the preferred date.

The ECHCS Director needs to ensure that scheduling staff use the clinically indicated or preferred appointment date when scheduling primary care patient appointments.

Specialty Care Appointments

For 25 of the 150 consults reviewed, schedulers used the providers' clinically indicated date annotated in the consult referral notes instead of the earliest appropriate date shown on the consult referral. The dates used by the scheduler were 2 to 6 weeks in the future. VHA's Directive 2010-027, *VHA Outpatient Scheduling Processes and Procedures*, June 9, 2010, does not use the terminology clinically indicated date but generally states that in conjunction with the provider's specified date the patient establishes a desired date of care.

In March 2015, VHA issued guidance for consult procedures stating the ordering provider must enter a date into the earliest appropriate date field to show the provider's clinically indicated date. Although the sample we reviewed included consults prior to March 2015, the sample consults included the earliest appropriate date and clinically indicated date terminology. To conduct our evaluation, we used the March 2015 guidance to supplement VHA Directive 2010-027.

We also consulted the co-chair of the VHA Consult Steering Committee who helped create the consult management directive and guidance for clarification. He told us that the earliest appropriate date on the consult referral is considered the clinically indicated date and ordering providers could set this date in the future if clinically appropriate. He further stated that providers should not routinely use a future clinically indicated date for new patient consults due to a lack of access or as a form of triage. He reviewed three examples from our review and stated that, since there was no clinical rationale for scheduling the new patient appointments several weeks out into the future, the use of the provider's future date was inappropriate. For example, if a patient needs to start on a new medication or needs a follow-up study before seeing the specialty provider, this may be an appropriate clinical rationale for scheduling a consult in the future.

Example 2 illustrates the improper use of the future clinically indicated date.

Example 2

A primary care provider requested a neurology consult on December 4, 2014, which was also the earliest appropriate date for scheduling an appointment. The provider entered a future appointment date of up to 4 weeks from the referral date on the consult. On December 10, 2014, staff scheduled the veteran's appointment for January 26, 2015, using January 4, 2015, as the clinically indicated date, which was just over 4 weeks from the referral date. While the veteran waited for the appointment 53 days from the December 4th referral date, the HAS Chief stated this veteran was not on the VCL because staff's use of the inappropriate clinically indicated date resulted in the appointment only showing a 22-day wait time.

The ECHCS Director needs to ensure that scheduling staff use the earliest appropriate date when scheduling new patient appointments.

VCL Was Not Accurate

For 229 of the 288 veterans with appointments over 30 days, NVCC staff did not add 173 veterans to the VCL in a timely manner and they did not add 56 veterans to the list at all. The NVCC Manager stated that, on a daily basis, NVCC staff should identify veterans who are waiting more than 30 days for their appointment. NVCC staff should then add the veterans to the VCL so the VCP contractors can coordinate the veterans' care with outside providers.

Veterans Not Timely Added to VCL

The NVCC staff did not add 173 veterans to the VCL in a timely manner. When VHA first implemented VCP, NVCC staff were unclear on how the process should work and did not conduct daily reviews to identify all veterans who had been waiting more than 30 days for their appointment. Examples 3 and 4 highlight the delay associated with adding veterans to the VCL.

Example 3

On January 15, 2015, a primary care provider requested an audiology consult for a veteran, which was also the clinically indicated date for scheduling an appointment. On February 4, 2015, Audiology staff scheduled an appointment for the veteran for April 15, 2015, which resulted in a wait time of 90 days. NVCC staff added the veteran to the VCL on March 26, 2015. The HAS Chief agreed that the veteran should have been added to the VCL on February 4, 2015.

Example 4

CBOC staff completed a veteran's initial enrollment on December 12, 2014, with the disposition as "SCHEDULE FUTURE EXAM." On December 12, 2014, primary care staff scheduled a primary care appointment for the veteran for January 26, 2015, resulting in a wait time of 45 days. NVCC staff added the veteran to the VCL on January 14, 2015. The HAS Chief agreed that NVCC staff should have added the veteran to the VCL on December 12, 2014.

Veterans Not On the VCL

For 56 of the 229 appointments, the NVCC Manager inadvertently omitted the CBOCs when identifying veterans who were waiting more than 30 days for their appointment. When identifying appointments scheduled to occur more than 30 days beyond the clinically indicated or preferred appointment date, the NVCC Manager only reviewed appointments scheduled at the VAMC Denver. Once we brought the issue to the HAS Chief's attention, he worked with the NVCC Manager to correct the VCL to include eligible veterans from the CBOCs. As of March 23, 2015, the NVCC manager had added 2,338 new veterans to the VCL. The ECHCS Director needs to ensure that staff places all veterans in ECHCS with appointments waiting over 30 days on the VCL within 1 day of scheduling the appointment.

CBOC Staff Did Not Timely Process Consults and Appointments

CBOC staff did not timely process 94 consults and primary care appointment requests, which contributed to appointment delays. For 28 of the 54 consults with appointments that CBOC staff scheduled beyond 30 days of the clinically indicated or preferred appointment date, they did not act upon the consult within 7 days. According to the Consult Business Management Rules, consults are placed in pending status when they are created, and staff must change the consult status within 7 days to reflect the appropriate action. Those actions include discontinued, canceled, scheduled, or completed.

Example 5 describes the untimely processing of a consult request.

Example 5

A primary care provider made a consult referral to Optometry Service on October 22, 2014, which was also the clinically indicated date for scheduling an appointment. Optometry staff did not acknowledge receipt of this request until December 23, 2014. Then, on December 30, 2014, Optometry staff scheduled an appointment for the referred veteran for December 31, 2014, which was 69 days after the clinically indicated date.

For the 234 primary care appointments that CBOC staff scheduled beyond 30 days of the clinically indicated or preferred appointment date, 66 were for newly enrolled veterans who requested an appointment. We contacted the team lead for VHA's Access and Clinic Administration Program who stated that appointment requests for newly enrolled veterans should be processed within a day, if not immediately. These 66 appointments were not scheduled for an average of 51 days after the appointment request date— ranging from 9 to 156 days.

Example 6 depicts the untimely action to process and schedule a primary care appointment.

Example 6

CBOC staff completed a veteran's enrollment on August 18, 2014, with the disposition to "SCHEDULE FUTURE EXAM." On November 4, 2014, or 78 days later, CBOC staff scheduled a primary care appointment for the veteran for January 6, 2015.

The HAS Chief told us that these delays occurred because, despite a high volume of consults and new patient appointment requests, the CBOC has a limited number of administrative staff available for processing the consults and scheduling appointments. The ECHCS Director needs to ensure that resources are sufficient for staff to act on consults within 7 days, and appointment requests for newly enrolled veterans within 1 day of the approved appointment request.

Conclusion

We substantiated the allegation that Colorado Springs veterans did not receive timely care in the Audiology, Mental Health, Neurology, Optometry, Orthopedic, and Primary Care Services. We determined that staff did not add veterans to the VCL as required. This was due to scheduling staff's use of incorrect clinically indicated or preferred appointment dates when scheduling appointments and failure of NVCC staff to properly manage the VCL by not ensuring veterans were added to the list in a timely manner. In addition, CBOC staff did not timely act on consults and new patient appointment requests. As a result, VA staff did not fully use Veterans Choice Program funds to afford Colorado Springs CBOC veterans the opportunity to receive timely care.

Recommendations

1. We recommended the Eastern Colorado Health Care System Director ensure that scheduling staff use the clinically indicated or preferred appointment dates when scheduling primary care patient appointments.

2. We recommended the Eastern Colorado Health Care System Director ensure that scheduling staff use the earliest appropriate date when scheduling new patient appointments.

3. We recommended the Eastern Colorado Health Care System Director ensure that staff place all veterans with appointments occurring over 30 days after the clinically indicated or preferred appointment date on the Veterans Choice List within 1 day of scheduling the appointment.

4. We recommended the Eastern Colorado Health Care System Director ensure that resources are sufficient for scheduling staff to act on consults within 7 days and appointment requests for newly enrolled veterans within 1 day of the approved appointment request.

Management Comments

The acting director of the ECHCS concurred in principle with our recommendations. The acting director acknowledged that staff who scheduled appointments were not 100 percent compliant with scheduling policies, but did not agree with OIG's retroactive application of the March 2015 VHA Interim Consult standard operating procedures to consults that staff created prior March 2015. ECHCS staff reported they have initiated a number of corrective actions to become compliant with current VHA scheduling guidance. ECHCS installed new clinic leadership and has taken action to train schedulers and ensure compliance with scheduling procedures and the use of appropriate clinically indicated or preferred appointment dates. In addition, ECHCS has taken action to ensure staff entered all veterans eligible for VCP on the VCL, and replaced and added staff to help ensure staff meet VHA scheduling protocols at the Colorado Springs outpatient clinic.

OIG Response

The acting director's planned corrective actions are acceptable. The acting director noted that prior to March 2015 ECHCS had no guidance on the use of the earliest appropriate date field on the consult request. However, VHA has had guidance for a number of years over the management of consults. Although the March 2015 VHA Interim Consult standard operating procedures made some changes, VHA's policy has always been to complete clinical consults consistent with VHA timeliness standards and individual health care needs. We do not believe the March 2015 VHA Interim Consult standard operating procedures changed that intent.

Based on corrective actions already implemented, we consider Recommendation 1 closed. We will monitor the facility's progress and follow up on the implementation of the remaining recommendations until all proposed actions are completed. Appendix C provides the full text of the ECHCS Acting Director's comments.

Appendix A   Background

Access, Choice, and Accountability Act of 2014

To improve veterans' access to timely medical care, Congress passed VACAA on August 7, 2014. This act became Public Law 113-146 when the President signed it on the same day. VACAA directs VA to establish a program to furnish hospital care and medical services through non-VA health care providers to veterans who either cannot be seen within VHA wait-time goals, or who qualify based on their place of residence more than 40 miles from a VA medical facility. VHA initiated the VCP in response to VACAA in November 2014.

This program allowed staff to identify veterans to include on the VCL, a list that includes veterans with appointments beyond 30 days from the clinically indicated or preferred appointment dates and veterans who live more than 40 miles from a VA facility. Under VCP, VA facilities began providing non-VA care to eligible veterans enrolled in VA health care as of August 1, 2014, and to recently discharged combat veterans who are within 5 years of their post—combat separation date. Congress authorized VCP to continue until the date the VCP funds are exhausted, or until August 7, 2017, whichever occurs first.

Effective June 8, 2015, VA implemented the Choice First process that incorporates a VCP option earlier in the referral hierarchy when care is not available within VA facilities or the facility cannot meet VHA timeliness standards. The new hierarchy is as follows:

- Refer the veteran to another facility. The referring facility may use existing Department of Defense, Indian Health Service facilities, and Tribal organizations agreements to get the veteran care.

- Refer the veteran to VCP when the program covers the needed services.

- Use other non-VA care options if VCP does not cover the needed services.

Veterans Choice Implementation

To fulfill the VCP mission, VHA implemented procedures for medical facilities to establish a VCL. The facilities need to identify and include new and established patients on the VCL who have waited more than 30 days from the clinically indicated or preferred appointment date, or reside more than 40 miles from a VA facility.

VA staff mail letters to eligible veterans and the veterans choose whether to receive the services outside VA facilities by contacting one of the VCP contractors using a phone number provided in the letter. To ensure eligible veterans could obtain services when they called, the contract terms state VA will provide daily updates to the VCL for veterans who are eligible because they have been waiting more than 30 days for their appointment and weekly updates for veterans meeting the 40-mile eligibility rule. VA amended the

40-mile straight-line calculation to use the distance the veteran must travel to the nearest VA medical facility via a mapped route on April 24, 2015.

Appendix B   Scope and Methodology

We conducted our review from February through October 2015. Our focus for the services in question was on the CBOC Colorado Springs consult processing and appointment scheduling during fiscal year 2015.

We examined applicable national and local policies, procedures, and guidance related to the VACAA, VCP, VCL, consult processing, and appointment scheduling. We conducted interviews with key CBOC and VAMC staff members and leadership with relevant knowledge or insight. We obtained and analyzed consult and appointment data to determine if the CBOC and VAMC staff acted on consult requests within 7 days, and scheduled appointments within 30 days of clinically indicated or preferred appointment dates of care. We reviewed audiology, mental health, optometry, neurology, and orthopedic consults and primary care appointments to determine if staff met the consult processing and appointment scheduling requirements. We also reviewed and identified veterans who were on the VCL and determined when staff added the veterans to the list.

To determine whether staff scheduled appointments for specialty care within 30 days of the clinically indicated or preferred appointment dates or added the patients to the VCL in a timely manner, we reviewed randomly selected non-statistical samples of 30 referrals for Audiology, Mental Health, Neurology, Optometry, and Orthopedic Services. These specialty consults were either in a completed, active, or pending status. The following table shows the universe of consults, the number of consults reviewed, and the dates we identified the consults.

Table 2. Number of Consults by Specialty in 2015

Specialty	Number of Consults	Number Reviewed	Date We Identified the Consults
Audiology	582	30	February 23
Mental Health	531	30	April 28
Neurology	1,473	30	April 28
Optometry	1,943	30	April 9
Orthopedic	2,909	30	April 28

Source: OIG Analysis of VHA Support Service Center Consult Data

To determine whether staff scheduled appointments for primary care within 30 days of the clinically indicated or preferred appointment dates, or added the patients to the VCL in a timely manner, we reviewed 300 of

2,246 primary care appointments completed during December 2014 and January 2015.

Data Reliability

We used computer-processed data from VHA Support Service Center's Consult Cube and Wait Time Final Cube. To assess the reliability of Consult Cube data, we compared consult request and completion date information reported in the cube, for Audiology, Mental Health, Neurology, Optometry, and Orthopedic services, with the Compensation and Pension Records Interchange consult data to ensure that the dates reported in the Consult Cube were supported. We were able to review enough consults to sufficiently rely on data from the Consult Cube for our conclusions. To assess the reliability of Wait Time Final Cube data, we compared appointment create date and appointment date information reported in the cube for primary care appointments with Computerized Patient Record System appointment data to ensure that the dates reported in the Wait Time Final Cube were supported. We were able to review enough appointments to determine the information was reliable for our conclusions.

Government Standards

We conducted this review in accordance with the *Quality Standards for Inspection and Evaluation* published by the Council of Inspectors General on Integrity and Efficiency.

Appendix C   Eastern Colorado Health Care System Director Comments

Department of Veterans Affairs   **Memorandum**

Date: December 22, 2015

From: Acting Director, VA Eastern Colorado Health Care System (554/00)

Subj: Draft Report, Review of Alleged Untimely Care at the Colorado Springs Community Based Outpatient Clinic. Project Number 2015-02472-R5-0133

To: Assistant Inspector General for Audits and Evaluations (52)

Thru: Director, Rocky Mountain Network (10N/19)

This Memorandum is in response to the Draft Report for the review of Alleged Untimely Care at the Colorado Springs Community Based Outpatient Clinic as referenced. Eastern Colorado Health Care System (ECHCS) is providing a response to each allegation and recommendation as instructed in your Memorandum of October 29, 2015. Overall, ECHCS agrees, in principle, with the recommendations provided. As of the date of this response, ECHCS has executed a substantial number of corrective actions to become compliant, and sustain compliance, with current VHA scheduling guidance, as noted below.

ECHCS does not concur with the retroactive application of the March 2015 VHA Interim Consult SOP to ECHCS consults created months prior to the release of that SOP. Retroactive application of national guidance for the specialty care appointment findings on page 4 of the draft report is a flawed methodology, at its foundation.

Recommendation 1: We recommended the Eastern Colorado Health Care System Director ensure that scheduling staff use the correct clinically indicate date or preferred appointment date when scheduling primary care patient appointments.

Target Date for Completion: December 30, 2015.

Facility Response: Concur, with additional comments

Eastern Colorado acknowledges that staff who scheduled appointments at the Colorado Springs Community Based Outpatient Clinic (CBOC) between December 2014 and January 2015 were not 100% compliant in following the clinically indicated date or patient preferred date. Under new clinic leadership, the following additional actions have been taken over the last eleven months to ensure scheduling compliance in Colorado Springs:

Analysis/Organizational Structure – Supervisory review conducted between December 2014 and January 2015 resulted in removal/replacement of a clinical manager, restructuring of the Colorado Springs clinic, and realignment of all scheduling staff under the Health Administrative Service. Additional actions taken included: establishment of an interim on-sight executive level leader, selection of a permanent on-sight, executive level leader, and recruitment of multiple key positions including, two Administrative Officers, three scheduling supervisors, 16 new schedulers, two scheduling trainers, three scheduling leads, and two Patient Advocates. Current facility leadership, in consultation with Human Resources, is determining whether administrative actions are warranted for individuals involved.

Expectations/Tools –Standard scheduling processes were established during Primary Care and Specialty Care rapid process improvement scheduling workshops, which resulted in standard processes and scripts, an electronic scheduling handbook (published in July 2015) and staff retraining. Selection of a new Health Administration (HAS) Chief in late January 2015, focused efforts on increasing completion of scheduling audits (12 per scheduler per month) which resulted in an increase of completed audits from 15% to 100%.

Recommendation 2: We recommended the Eastern Colorado Health Care System Director ensure that scheduling staff use the earliest appropriate appointment date when scheduling new patient appointments.

Target Date for Completion: Complete

ECHCS Comment: Concur that ECHCS should follow VHA guidance in relation to use of the Earliest Appropriate Date (EAD). ECHCS does not concur with retroactive application of VHA guidance released months after the creation of the 25 consults cited on page 4 of the report under Specialty Care Appointments.

OIG reviewed 25 consults dated from December 2014 through January 2015, where providers set clinically indicated dates on the consult that were 2 to 6 weeks in the future, based on the referring provider's clinical judgement. Schedulers then used the provider's clinically indicated date to schedule appointments appropriately. The verbiage on page 4, Specialty Care Appointments section (first paragraph, second sentence) infers that schedulers used the clinically indicated date from the provider to intentionally misrepresent the wait time. This is not an accurate reflection of the work performed as the scheduler was appropriately scheduling from the provider's CID. In addition and for clarification purposes, on page 5, Example 2, when the Health Administration Chief stated that the Veteran was not on the VCL due to the scheduler using an inappropriate CID, that statement was made based upon the newly released VHA Interim Consult SOP. It was not based upon accepted practices at the time the specialty care consults in question were created and scheduled.

The "Interim Consult SOP" released in March 2015 provided guidance that the CID should be entered into the Earliest Appropriate Date (EAD) field, but did not provide guidance on how to set a CID. The VHA Consult Steering Committee, as cited in the OIG report, began providing guidance after the SOP was released to providers. That guidance was to set the day the referring provider identified a clinical need, as the CID, unless a medically indicated reason was documented in the consult. This guidance was not in effect at the time the consults in question were created and scheduled. The VHA Access and Clinic Administration Program Office confirmed that official guidance was not provided, in relation to entering into the EAD field, before March 2015. In the absence of specific official guidance, it was acceptable practice for a provider to use the date they determined to be clinically appropriate. That resulted in a range of dates due to patient specific, clinical determinations by Primary Care and Specialty Care providers.

After the March 2015 SOP was released to the field, ECHCS trained all schedulers on the use of CID and EAD. In October 2015, ECHCS completed 100% scheduling audit. All schedulers in Colorado Springs have demonstrated competency in using

CID (now EAD field) on consults. Based upon audit results, scheduling supervisors and trainers are continuously providing feedback to schedulers and retraining them as necessary.

Recommendation 3: We recommended the Director of the Eastern Colorado Health Care System ensure that all veterans with appointments occurring over 30 days after the clinically indicated date or preferred appointment date are placed on the Veterans Choice List within 1 day of scheduling the appointment.

Target Date for Completion: Complete

ECHCS Comment: Concur, with additional comments

At the time of this review, the VHA did not have a standard report or a process developed to identify appointments eligible to be added to the Veterans Choice List (VCL), or a requirement to add them to the VCL in one business day. VA facilities were instructed to develop local processes. A process was developed locally based upon information available at the time.

The employee responsible for obtaining the report of patients eligible to place on the VCL incorrectly ran a report, which excluded some of our sites of care, Colorado Springs CBOC being one of them. When this was identified in April 2015, the affected patients were immediately placed on the VCL. The employee was counseled and retrained on how to run the VCL report to include all sites of care in ECHCS. At the time of this review through the time of this response, VHA has not provided a report to identify patients with appointments occurring more than 30 days after the clinically indicated or patient preferred date who were not added to the VCL.

Of note, Phase III of the Choice Program will transition the eligibility portion of the process from the VCL to another process entirely. This process requires uploading of an eligibility form into the Health Net software, DOMA, for all eligible patients that opt-in to this benefit. ECHCS has assigned this task to four Medical Support Assistants in the local Non-VA Care Coordination/Choice team, with oversight from the new Choice Program Administrator.

Recommendation 4: We recommended the Eastern Colorado Health Care System Director ensure that resources are sufficient for scheduling staff to act on consults within 7 days and appointment requests for newly enrolled veterans within 1 day.

Target Date for Completion: April 30, 2016

ECHCS Comment: Concur, with additional comments

ECHCS is committed to appropriately scheduling newly enrolled veterans timely, although ECHCS does not concur with retroactive application of a policy that wasn't in place when the appointments were scheduled or at the time of the OIG audit.

This location experienced a 13.3% unique patient increase between FY14 and FY15, which is among the highest of any VHA facility in the country. During the time period reviewed, the clinic had just consolidated three locations into one 80,000 square foot clinic, had significant key position vacancies (including schedulers, Patient Advocate, Administrative Officers, CBOC Manager, Nurse Manager), was attempting to operationalize a call center without additional staff, and had an ineffective scheduler and CBOC supervisory structure. These facts contributed to the Colorado Springs Outpatient Clinic scheduling challenges during December 2014 and January 2015.

In response ECHCS has taken the following staffing actions from April through September 2015 to meet the challenges of the Colorado Springs Outpatient Clinic: replacement of a clinical manager, selection of a permanent on-sight, executive level leader, two Administrative Officers, HAS section chief responsible for all Chief Business Office functions, three scheduling supervisors, two scheduling trainers, three scheduling leads, 16 new schedulers, and two Patient Advocates. The new management infrastructure and new staff will ensure VHA scheduling protocols are met going forward and ECHCS will maintain a minimum of 85% scheduling audit completion rate for FY16.

(original signed by:)

Cory B. Ramsey, RN, MHA, NEA-BC
Acting Director

Approve/Disapprove

(Original signed by:)

Ralph Gigliotti
Network Director, VISN 19

GentilucciT: 11/5/15_____OI_____OO

Appendix D   OIG Contact and Staff Acknowledgments

OIG Contact	For more information about this report, please contact the Office of Inspector General at (202) 461-4720.
Acknowledgments	Larry Reinkemeyer, Director Josh Belew Robin Frazier Ken Myers

Appendix E   Report Distribution

VA Distribution

Office of the Secretary
Veterans Health Administration
Veterans Benefits Administration
National Cemetery Administration
Assistant Secretaries
Office of General Counsel

Non-VA Distribution

House Committee on Veterans' Affairs
House Appropriations Subcommittee on Military Construction,
   Veterans Affairs, and Related Agencies
House Committee on Oversight and Government Reform
Senate Committee on Veterans' Affairs
Senate Appropriations Subcommittee on Military Construction,
   Veterans Affairs, and Related Agencies
Senate Committee on Homeland Security and Governmental Affairs
National Veterans Service Organizations
Government Accountability Office
Office of Management and Budget
U.S. Senate: Michael F. Bennet, Cory Gardner
U.S. House of Representatives: Ken Buck, Mike Coffman, Diana DeGette,
   Doug Lamborn, Ed Perlmutter, Jared Polis, Scott Tipton

www.ingramcontent.com/pod-product-compliance
Lightning Source LLC
Chambersburg PA
CBHW080535190526

45169CB00008B/3177